Dora's Anti-Aging Guide

LaDore Labs

http://ladore.me

Dora @ LaDore Labs

Table Of Content

- Introduction. Skin-deep or life-deep? - 3
- Common Sense Anti-Aging - 6
- The One – Anti-Aging Secret - 8
- Skin Care ROUTINE – Daily Regimen - 16
- Mini-facial - 20
- Homemade Anti-Aging Scrub - 21
- Anti-Aging Masques - 24
- Vaseline For Wrinkles - Myth or Reality? - 29
- Basic Homemade Recipes - 33
-   6 Cleansers
-   Toners
-   Moisturizers
-   Spot Treatment
- Ingredients in the recipes - 35
- Examples of incorrectly applied homemade solutions - 37
- How I Anti-Wrinkled My Mother-In-Law - 39

Introduction. Skin-deep or life-deep?

From becoming aware of the dissonance:
"In my head, I'm still 20."
"Oh no, is this me?"

To skin-deep concerns:
"I am not looking forward to wrinkles. I don't want
to get wrinkles too quickly."
"I'm worried about losing my looks and feeling the
pressure of my age."
"Is my face sagging?"
"I know my looks are gonna start to deteriorate."
"Wrinkles, wrinkles, more wrinkles... Sigh..."

To life-deep concerns:
"Suddenly, I've realized that aging is the younger
cousin of dying."
"The wrinkles and the double chin are smoke
screens for what we're really afraid of - mortality..."

The prospect of losing my looks fills me with such
crushing dread. I start taking care of myself.
Finally, healthy lifestyle and plenty sunscreen.

But deep inside I know that I am powerless to stop
getting older. As we grow older, the inexorable
march of wrinkles and grey hair reminds us of our
own waning power.

We've been trained by the society not to notice

wisdom and experience, rather weakness and ugliness. So when the inevitable truth of aging confronts us in a mirror – we don't react well. The ultimate compliment has become, "Oh, you don't look your age!" Age has become a disease, to be cured and eradicated.

Of course, before anything, before you even think of skincare and Anti-Aging - reframe yourself. Give it time and effort, it's well worth it. How?

Getting old is just another part of the exciting process of life. You gain experience, wisdom, understanding. You build internal beauty, refining your personality, developing precious character traits missing in younger age. Perhaps, you are getting more than enough compensation for deteriorating your looks?

But don't take reframing as a pill. It's not a pill. It's truth.

At the same time, be alert. If you gain wrinkles too many, and too deep, before you gain enough wisdom and experience to make up for your elusive external beauty - you are in trouble.

This is exactly where anti-aging skincare can help. It cannot stop time, neither it can reverse it. But it can slow it down for you, minimize your lines, reduce your wrinkles, restore your skin's youth and beauty to the greatest extent possible, and... Use the time to acquire wisdom, wisdom, and more wisdom, build your internal beauty. So when you reach the point when no skincare can possibly help any more, you won't even notice it, because at that point the polished surface won't be of essence...

Common Sense Anti-Aging

Many changes take place when we become older.

1. Cells divide much slower. Skin becomes thin and fragile.
2. Less oil is produced, thus dryer skin, age spots, and wrinkles.
3. Collagen and elastin production slows down. Elasticity, tone, and texture suffer; wrinkles and fine lines appear.
4. Cells containing pigment decrease, thus age spots and liver spots appear.
5. The fat layer is getting lost, so the fat moves and resettles, creating bags under the eyes and saggy skin.
6. Blood vessels become fragile, thus broken capillaries and bleeding become common.
7. Changes in bone and muscle take place, thus saggy skin.

These seven fundamental changes have one underlying cause. The main cause is believed to be the damage done by free radicals. It is still a theory, not a fact, but it's well substantiated theory. It was proposed in 1950s, and plenty evidence has been found since then.

Based on this fact, we can formulate our Common Sense Anti-Aging approach. There will be two branches:

1. Not letting free radicals in. I call it border patrol.
2. Fight off those free radicals already in. I call it antioxidant therapy.

You are under free radicals' attack if you are:

- Exposed to sunrays
- Exposed to cigarette smoke
- Lack sleep
- Under stress
- Sadness
- In a toxic environment
- Using toxic household products
- Having a poor diet
- Consume alcohol excessively
- Use harsh soaps

These are common examples. Avoid, prevent, stay away from these – and your aging will slow down considerably.

And what about antioxidants? Where are they coming from? Correct, from good healthy diet!

That's all on common sense anti-aging. Don't underestimate simplicity. Having the basic framework, you can fill the gaps with what you already know, and make quite a difference.

The One – Anti-Aging Secret

I get this question from time to time. In fact, this is my favorite question. The beginning of the question varies, these are just some examples:

- I am overwhelmed
- I have no time
- I have no money
- My mom never did it, why should I

and the end of the question boils down to:

I will use only one product, what should it be?

This is indeed a great question, because it compels to establish priorities. In an extensive array of products - what's the most important, crucial, number one? What is The One?

As I am focusing on anti-aging, I am talking about women over 30 years old. The answer for younger women and girls would be different.

Introducing The One (....drum-roll....): A Night Cream.

Let me tell you a story which is many years old... Very many years old... Once upon a time I came to this country, leaving behind Asia and Europe. I graduated pharmacy school for the second time (the first time was on another continent) and opened my pharmacy. For the first few months I was rebellious: I called the doctors back yelling at them, demanding them to explain why in the world they want this patient to take this medicine if the patient can get cured by lemon, garlic, chicken soup, cayenne, turmeric, sea salt, fresh air, a few days on a beach, and by other "medicines", more or less exotic but still very natural. Unsuccessful in my war against medical establishment, I quickly gave up, and established a large natural section in my pharmacy. Vitamins, supplements, herbs, thousands of titles from hundreds of brands, from all over the world.

My favorite visitors were girls and women with skin concerns. After all this was my area of expertise for many years already. The faces got cleared, perfected, beautified, and more and more local women walked in in a quest for beauty.

How did I handle women with Anti-Wrinkle inquiries and Anti-Aging concerns? Well, you have to realize the subtlety of the moment. Here I am, unusually looking woman with a strange accent of unknown origin, wanting so much to help a suffering customer, to give her the gift of beautiful skin, but worrying about a customer spending too much money on the way.

I tried countless combinations of countless cheap

products, discovered the companies making simple yet quality stuff, and composed unique regimens for my dear clients. But not everything could be replaced cheaply without compromising results. One product I refused to compromise and substitute for a cheaper alternative. It had to be the best one. It was the Night Cream! Because it's the crucial product, the game changer.

Number one

My flagship product – the night cream - supplemented with cheap (but quality) products worked wonders. The "cheap" supplementation was quite a challenge, I would say it was arduous work to select the right products.

That's when I became a chef again – I started cooking my own flagship product, the night cream, as it had to be best of the best. The flagship product was the main player, providing advanced anti-aging action, and other products were meant to be supportive, to produce no harm, and to give at least some minimal benefits.

To those who were willing to try, I gave wonderful homemade recipes. That is, except for a night cream. There are no shortcuts for a night cream.

Number two

What if I tell you that you could amplify the efficiency of a night cream many times over? Such an amplifier would be number two, after a night cream.

The amplifier is (.... drum-roll....): A Serum!

How does a serum amplify the action?

First of all, let's understand the serums better. A serum contains the most potent dose of anti-aging ingredients comparing to any other skincare product, including a night cream. Due to a high concentration and huge quantity of active ingredients a serum may be more expensive than other products. However, you usually need a tiny amount, so even a small jar should last for months. By their very nature serums are extremely efficient in what they are designed to achieve. To compound the efficiency, serums are made of small molecules, thus the active ingredients are absorbed by the skin quicker and deeper than anything else, including the best moisturizers.

Let me put it this way: a night cream is a moisturizer with benefits, while a serum is benefits without a moisturizer (this statement is not precise, as serum's benefits may also include deep moisturizing action, yet the statement conveys the essence of a serum very well). By the way, that's exactly why it makes no sense to use a serum without a moisturizer - the skin will not look and feel right. A moisturizer and a serum complement each other and as a couple generate the benefits significantly higher that a sum of their respective benefits if taken alone.

About eye cream

The skin around eyes has plenty in common with the rest of the facial skin. In fact, in many countries with advanced skincare there was no such a thing as an eye cream at all for a long time. Why not?

Because your night cream is also good for the skin around your eyes.

However, when it comes to aging, the skin around the eyes has certain unique properties. Yes, there is wrinkling and sagging, but there are also distinct phenomena as puffiness, dark circles, crow's feet, etc. Regular moisturizer is not designed to deal with special eye-area related issues. Moisturizer is good indeed, but not enough in the eye area. Things also get complicated by the eye area skin being very thin.

A good eye cream is a combination product: it's somewhat in between serum and moisturizer. It's more serum than moisturizer, and it's more moisturizer than serum. Its molecules are much smaller than those of regular moisturizer. It's packed with large amounts of active ingredients, just like serum is,- those a good moisturizer has, plus those responsible for unique aging signs around the eyes.

If you already have a serum and a moisturizer – you can use them both, as a combination, around the eyes, that's the best approximation of an eye cream! In fact, that's what an eye cream is, by a large extent. That's why it's more expensive than a moisturizer, because it's more like a serum, contains huge amount of active ingredients. At the same time, you need very little amount of it to be applied each time, so it should last longer, just like a serum.

So you have two options: 1) use your regular moisturizer under your eyes (if more sensitive skin in the eye area takes it gracefully), or 2) use a night cream AND a serum.

If You Don't Do THIS - Nothing Else Matters

If you don't do THIS - then even the fanciest, most expensive, and most efficient skincare products are waste of time. Almost literally. Now guess: what is THIS?

A good moisturizer is designed to penetrate the skin, supplying the skin with good stuff. However, it's not easy to penetrate the skin. There is an obstacle on the way. What is it? A layer of dead skin cells. Such a layer of dead skin cells is not really bad news per se. But it's bad news for a moisturizer, especially good quality one. Because dead cells block it from being able to penetrate the skin. Any moisturizer under such circumstances will be ineffective, and essentially waste of money. And not only a moisturizer, for that matter.

Thus exfoliating is not an option, it's a MUST. Exfoliating takes off the dead skin cells, gets rid of the debris clogging your pores, and allows moisturizer and other skincare products to do their job.

Excellent exfoliating option would be going to the ocean and spending a week or two swimming and sunbathing daily. Just be careful with overdoing the sun. By the way, absolutely no swimming pools, swimming pool would make it worse. Warm water and hot sand can prepare your skin for the very best skincare of your choice.

Another exfoliating option would be visiting a sauna. Especially combined with a good scrub right there, but even without a scrub a sauna may make quite a difference.

And, of course, your exfoliator, or a scrub.

Sufficiently exfoliated skin may be easily

maintained. How often would you exfoliate routinely, using a scrub? Normally once a week. Sometimes twice a week. The weekly procedure is often called mini-facial, and exfoliation is a part of it.

The importance of exfoliation cannot be overstated. It's crucial. Nothing works to its full capacity without it.

Skin Care ROUTINE – Daily Regimen

P.M. Routine

- EYE MAKEUP REMOVER (if you have what to remove)
- CLEANSER
- MINI-FACIAL = {EXFOLIATOR, MASQUE} (once to twice a week)
- TONER or ASTRINGENT (if you are 30+)
- SERUM (if you are 35+) or CONCENTRATE (if you need to address specific issue that this concentrate is designed for)
- NIGHT CREAM
- Spot TREATMENT (if applicable)
- EYE CREAM

A.M. Routine

- WATER (no cleanser in the morning)
- TONER or ASTRINGENT (if you are 30+)
- SERUM (if you are 35+) or CONCENTRATE (in a case you need to address specific issue that this concentrate is designed for)
- DAY CREAM
- EYE CREAM (if you are 25+)
- SUNSCREEN (when applicable)
- MAKEUP (if any)

General skincare routine

- **Cleanser:** Apply with moistened hands, gently lather, then rinse. Stay away from the eyes. No cleanser in the morning, just wash with warm water.
- **Scrub** (first part of mini-facial; once or twice a week, as per the regimen): Rub it onto your face, covering all areas. Massage it in, using circular motions. Take about two minutes on your face. Remember to bring it down to your neck and chest. When done, wipe it off your skin using a clean cloth, or - better - rinse with warm water and then pat dry.
- **Anti-inflammatory [for oily skin]:** ICE therapy (to reduce redness and inflammation, usually applicable to the problem skin only)
- **Masque** (second part of mini-facial; once or twice a week, as per the regimen): Put on a face for 20-30 minutes. Stay away from the eyes. After 20-30 minutes wash with warm water.
- **Toner:** Apply to a cotton ball and gently wipe over your skin. Stay away from the eyes.
- **Serum:** pump some serum, gently put it on your face, and dab it. No rubbing! Dab it gently. To dab means to tap lightly. If you prefer to use both toner and serum, apply serum immediately after applying toner, while your skin is still wet.

- **Anti-inflammatory [for dry skin]:** ICE therapy (to reduce redness and inflammation, usually applicable to the problem skin only)
- **Moisturizer** (i.e. **night cream** or **day cream**): Dispense some amount of moisturizer on your hands. Apply the moisturizer to your skin (best if it's still dump after toner). Apply gently, do not rub vigorously. Stay away from the eyes (when needed, eyes prefer specialized moisturizer, an eye cream).
- **Spot Treatment:** Use a cotton swab to apply the treatment just on the pimple, or to the blemish - not on the surrounding area.
- Note: Ice is applied to problem skin to take off redness and inflammation. For oily skin this is done between scrub and masque, and on days with no mini-facial right after cleanser. For dry skin this is done right before night cream.

Your Skincare Routine is your most important asset for your skin. There is a lot of wisdom invested in it. This wisdom took centuries to develop.

Supplementation: Taking fish oil and acidophilus supplements is always very beneficial for the skin, but for dry skin and for problem skin supplementing with both fish oil and acidophilus is a must.

Mini-facial

Mini-facial is a procedure you do once or twice a week, as a part of your daily skincare routine, right after cleanser.

Mini-facial consists of two steps: 1) scrub, 2) masque. The terms "scrub" and "exfoliator" and "exfoliant" are synonymous.

I will present an amazingly effective anti-aging scrub, as well as an array of anti-aging masques. The masques will be many, for a good reason. Use them all, one at a time. Alternate them. Each masques focuses on certain anti-aging action, but together they provide everything your skin could dream about: vitamins, cleansing pores, tightening pores, toning the skin, making skin vibrant and clear, whitening, nourishing, hydrating, antioxidants, softening and clearing wrinkles, tightening the skin, helping to get rid of sagging skin, etc.

Mini-facial is a well kept secret to nearly miraculous results in Anti-Wrinkle in particular, and in skincare in general.

Homemade Anti-Aging Scrub

Anti-aging silver bullets are anti-aging moisturizer and serum. As they must penetrate the skin, delivering the active ingredients to the place of action, the skin has to be prepared. Exfoliation achieves just that. Here is the recipe of amazingly efficient scrub.

Ingredients.

- Baking Soda
- Coarse Almonds Flour (almonds coarsely blended)
- Milk (only whole milk, i.e. no reduce-fat, no low-fat, no skim milk)
- Water (filtered)
- Salt (quality sea salt)

For normal to oily skin:

Coarse Almonds Flour (1 teaspoon) +
Baking Soda (1 teaspoon) +
Salt (1 teaspoon) +
Water (1 teaspoon)
    = mix it all well, making into a paste

For normal to dry skin:

Coarse Almonds Flour (1 tablespoon) +
Baking Soda (1 teaspoon) +

Milk (1 teaspoon) +
Salt (a pinch)
   = mix it well, making into a paste.

Salt may be an irritant in some cases of dry skin. If that's the case, skip it.

Directions:

Put the paste on your face like a masque, covering all areas. Keep it on for 10 minutes. After 10 minutes massage it in, using circular motions (from the middle of a face to the sides – this is important, otherwise formation of wrinkles may be facilitated). Take about two minutes on your face. Remember to bring it down to your neck and chest. When done, wipe it off your skin using a clean cloth, or - better - rinse with warm water and then pat dry. If you have access to a steam room, spend the 10 minutes with the masque on your face right there; it will greatly enhance the action (steam room, not sauna with dry heat). Keep the scrub away from your eyes.

Results:

- A face becomes glowing
- Dead cells are removed
- Pores are cleansed and "breath" better
- Large pores become smaller
- Skin is no longer rough

- Skin becomes pleasantly thinner where necessary
- Skin is ready for subsequent application and penetration of the finest active ingredients

Anti-Aging Masques

11 Masques for normal to dry skin:

1. Turmeric (1 tsp) + Chickpea Flour (2 tblspn) + Milk (enough to form paste)
2. Avocado (1/2) + Egg Yolk (1) + Honey (1tsp)
3. Egg Yolk (1) + Honey (1 tsp) + Fine Almond Flour (enough to form paste)
4. Egg Yolk (1) + Honey (1 tsp) + Oatmeal Flour (enough to form paste)
5. Avocado (1/2) + Lemon (1/2) + Sour Cream (1 tsp) + Oatmeal Flour (enough to form paste)
6. [Cucumber (shredded, 1 tblspn) OR Banana (smashed, 1/2) OR Tomato (grated with no skin, 1/2)] + Fine Almond Flour (1 tblspn) + Sour Cream (1 tblspn)
7. {Banana (smashed, 1/3) + Heavy Cream (1 tsp)} - whip well, + Turmeric (1/2 tsp)
8. Farmers cheese (1 tblspn) + Vitamin E (1/2 tsp)
9. {Yeast (1 tsp) + Lemon Juice (1 tsp)} - whip, + Heavy Cream (approximately 1 tsp, enough to make paste) + 35% Hydrogen Peroxide (1-2 drops)
10. [Olive Oil (1 tsp) OR Coconut oil (1 tsp)] + Avocado (1/2) + [Banana (1/4) OR Peach (1) OR Strawberries (2)]
11. [Jojoba Oil (1 tsp) OR Almond Oil (1 tsp)] + [Papaya (2 tblspn) OR Cucumber (2 tblspn)]

+ Oatmeal Flour (approximately 1 tblspn, enough to make paste)

Hydrogen peroxide masque formula:

{LIQUID (1 tsp) + Yeast (1 tsp)} - whip,
+ Egg Yolk (1),
+ ADDITIVE (1 tsp),
+ 35% Hydrogen Peroxide (1-2 drops)

In this formula LIQUID and ADDITIVE are replaced by corresponding substances depending on a skin type as follows:

For dry skin: Liquid = Milk, Additive = Heavy Cream
For normal skin: Liquid = Water, Additive = Honey
For oily skin: Liquid = Lemon, Additive - none
For very oily skin with enlarged pores: Liquid = 3% Hydrogen Peroxide, Additive - none

For normal to oily skin:

Farmers Cheese (1 tblspn) +
Shredded Cucumber (1 tblspn) +
35% Hydrogen Peroxide (1-2 drops)

Manufacturing tip: in order for a masque to work properly the yeast should be completely dissolved in accompanying liquid.

Application tip: the masque may come out thicker or thinner, i.e. closer to thick paste, or closer to liquid. If it resembles liquid, use a brush to apply it layer after layer. Apply next layer when the previous layer dries out.

Usage tip: use the masque within a few minutes after you make it. It won't keep its properties if stored, even if refrigerated.

Directions:

Put on a face for 20-30 minutes. Stay away from the eyes. After 20-30 minutes wash with warm water.

You can also use a homemade masque unconventionally, i.e. whenever you are in a kitchen, coming across some good ingredients - just make an appropriate masque. Provided that you face is clean, washed with your favorite cleanser first.

Ingredients:

- [Fine] Almonds Flour: almonds blended well, till you have fine flour
- [Fine] Oatmeal Flour (or oat flour, just another term): oats (rolled or old-fashioned) finely blended
- Chickpea Flour: blended dried chickpeas, or

garbanzo beans. Also known as garbanzo flour, gram flour and besan.

- 3% hydrogen peroxide can be found in a local pharmacy.
- 35% hydrogen peroxide: search Amazon for "35% Food Grade Hydrogen Peroxide", you will see a few excellent options. Be careful to use only one to two drops of 35% hydrogen peroxide in any formula containing it as an ingredient, and exercise care when handling it, it's pretty strong. A tip: since you need 1-2 drops only, it would be convenient to first pour some amount into a dropper bottle.
- Yeast: this may be either dry yeast, or fresh yeast. It really depends on your preference, try it out to see what's easier for you to make, and which end result you like more. The key is to whip yeast with its accompanying liquid so that yeast would dissolve completely.
- Milk: whole milk (i.e. no reduce-fat, no low-fat, no skim milk)
- Lemon: freshly squeezed lemon juice. No notation: Lemon (1) means a whole squeezed lemon, i.e. juice squeezed from a whole lemon. Lemon (1/2) means half a lemon squeezed, i.e. juice squeezed from half a lemon. Lemon (1/2 tsp) and lemon (1 tsp) would mean half a teaspoon and one teaspoon of lemon juice respectively.
- Turmeric: powdered spice.

About flour:

You need coarse flour for your scrub, and fine flour for your masque. You can easily use a food processor or high rpm blender to make flour. Stop blending on time, before you flour is too fine in case you need it for a scrub. Fine flour will take just a bit longer.

Vaseline For Wrinkles - Myth or Reality?

There are two warring camps in the petroleum jelly debate. One camp advocates for petroleum jelly for everything, including wrinkles, while another camp outlaws Vaseline and is ready to impose a death penalty for its use.

There are cases when petroleum jelly is appropriate according to everyone. For example, in hot, dry desert, or for healing certain types of wounds, or in harsh cold weather. It has wonderful protective qualities. Putting petroleum jelly on your skin is like coating it in a layer of plastic.

What makes petroleum jelly attractive to be used in skincare?

1. It makes your skin softer
2. It retains moisture
3. It decreases fine lines on a face

Does it really? At least it seems that's what it does, but let's look closer.

1. It makes your skin feel softer, but does not actually make it softer. It does not change the quality of the skin. You feel the instant gratification of a softened surface.
2. It seals the moisture border: nothing will leave the skin, nothing will come in. This may

cause a range of problems. Something always has to leave, and something always has to come in. Skin has many functions, and sealing it off disrupts certain processes. Your skin is, in fact, suffocating, almost literally.

3. It only decreases appearance of fine lines, but not fine lines.

The benefits of petrolatum-based creams are in appearance only, in the way how the skin looks and feels. Such a cream does not correct or improve the skin. Moreover, talking long term consequences, the skin becomes saggy, loses its tone, pores may become enlarged, puffy eyes may result, you name it... Skin becomes old much earlier than it should, much faster than it would become otherwise.

Objectively there are plenty harmful consequences, but you can only call them harmful if you notice them. Otherwise there is no harm perceived. If you look in the mirror and are happy, so be it. Like the woman who recently wrote to me: "I have wrinkles and I worked hard to get them, so I'll wear them proudly."

The complexity of the processes in the skin cells is mind-boggling. Years ago we didn't know how to work with this complexity. So skincare was focused on a surface of the skin, on how it looks and feels. Petrolatum-based products served this concept well and did it cheaply. After all a byproduct of the oil industry is just plain cheap.

On the contrary, modern skin care technologies allow us to penetrate the skin, and to influence amazing processes in the skin. They work on a cell level.

Do you have to take advantage of those technologies? Not necessarily. It's up to you. You may well be okay with old-style products, they are still around, and they are not going away. Just be aware: anything based on petroleum jelly should be very cheap. If it's expensive – avoid it, the cheaper the better rule applies here.

Modern skin care just cannot be based on petroleum. Petrolatum will create tight plastic-like cover on your skin, and will sit on its surface. That's not what modern skincare is about.

In contrast, there are different kinds of carrier substances that have been discovered or created. Carriers will penetrate into the skin and carry active ingredients into the cells. Promoting cells longevity, boosting collagen, increased elastin production, blocking neurotransmitters responsible for wrinkle formation, anti-pigmentation effect, boosting skin repair and regeneration, just to name some benefits.

Looking back at petrolatum-based products, the

difference is staggering. The firmness and tone are improved; pigment spots and wrinkles are reduced; the size of pores is minimized; free radicals are neutralized. And the list goes on and on. Good old-fashioned creams never acted on this level altogether, they did nothing to the skin per se.

The choice is yours to make.

Basic Homemade Recipes

6 Cleansers

1. Raw milk (not pasteurized, not homogenized, not something-else-ized; this is the only "recipe" containing specifically raw milk)
2. Baking Soda + Jojoba Oil + Honey (equal amounts)
3. Tomato (1/2) + Lemon (1/2 tsp) + Milk (1 tsp)
4. Milk (1 tblspn) + Olive Oil (1 tsp) + Grapes Pulp (from 5-6 grapes)
5. Aloe Vera Leaf (peeled, take out 1 tblspn of gel-like mass) + Papaya (1 slice peeled and grated - approx 1 tblspn) + Honey (1 tblspn) + Yogurt (1 tblspn)
6. Cucumber (1/4, grated) + Yogurt (2tbl) + Cooked Oatmeal (2tbl) - this one is specifically for dry skin

Toners

1. **For oily skin:** Lemon juice (not for problem or irritated skin)
2. **For dry skin:** Lemon juice mixed with Water (not for problem or irritated skin)
3. **For all skin types:** Silver Water (for problem or irritated skin this is the only choice of a toner)
4. **For all skin types:** Apple Cider Vinegar +

Water (equal amounts)

Moisturizers

1. **For dry skin:** Jojoba Oil or Coconut Oil or Shea Butter or Cocoa Butter
2. **For oily skin:** Squalane Oil

A note on these two moisturizers. They are cheap and absolutely superior than any petroleum-based solution. But, of course, they don't do the advanced anti-aging action as a good professional moisturizer would do. This is not the case with scrubs and masques recipes. They are just as effective as the best commercial products. As for cleansers and toners, it really depends, you have to experiment.

Spot Treatment - for problem skin

1. Garlic
2. Zinc (2-3 caps) + Silver Water (enough to form paste)
3. Turmeric (1/4 tsp) + Toothpaste (1/2 tsp) + Zinc (1 cap)

Ingredients in the recipes

- Apple Cider Vinegar: Bragg's Organic Apple Cider Vinegar is a good option.
- Garlic: crushed and somewhat juiced garlic. Used as a spot treatment on a pimple.
- Lemon: freshly squeezed lemon juice. Lemon (1) means a whole squeezed lemon, i.e. juice squeezed from a whole lemon, Lemon (1/2) means half a lemon squeezed, i.e. juice squeezed from half a lemon. Lemon (1/2tsp) and lemon (1tsp) mean half a teaspoon and one teaspoon of lemon juice respectively.
- Simple Natural Toothpaste (this is not a brand name, this is just a simple and natural toothpaste). Has to be paste, not gel. Three ingredients are of interest to us: Calcium Carbonate, Sodium Bicarbonate, and Silica, everything else is of no essence, so the less other ingredients it contains, the better. Jason's toothpastes seem to be the best among a long list of toothpastes I've reviewed for this purpose. More specifically, Healthy Mouth® Tartar Control Toothpaste is perfect. It contains above mentioned ingredients, plus cinnamon and menthol, which are beneficial. Other Jason's toothpastes are also good, though this one is the best among them. If you get any other toothpaste, make sure it's paste and not gel, and avoid mint as an ingredient (peppermint

is okay, just mint shouldn't be there). Though off the subject, let's mention briefly that Jason's toothpastes seem to be the best for the teeth, not only for the skin, in terms of quality of their ingredients, the ingredients they have, and junky and toxic ingredients that they don't have. And just to mention a bit less than ideal names which would also work well: Powersmile® Whitening Toothpaste (not mint one), Sea Fresh® Strengthening Toothpaste, Nutrismile® Enamel Defense Toothpaste. Please note: for the reasons beyond our scope here, it should be specifically toothpaste, and nothing else. The same ingredients taken in powdered form and mixed will not work at all.

- Turmeric: spice powder.
- Zinc: specifically zinc supplement. Either open a capsule, or crush a tablet. Chelated might be beneficial, copper as an added ingredient is a plus, but neither is a must, as long as it's zinc supplement. Zinc (1cap) and zinc (3caps) means the powder from one zinc supplement capsule and from three capsules respectively. One capsule may contain 25mg – 50gm of zinc, but this really doesn't matter.

Examples of incorrectly applied homemade solutions

- Garlic can be used as spot treatment only. Used on a whole face may burn the skin, while as a spot treatment it's just great when needed.
- Honey is good in certain situations, but it shouldn't be applied on irritated skin. Also, watch out for allergy on honey.
- Also, honey may be a wrong remedy for another reason in case of acne. Acne may be of bacterial origin, and may be of fungal origin. Honey acts as an antibiotic and inhibits bacteria (especially manuka honey). At the same time fungus loves honey, so if you use honey while having fungus-related acne, then you are asking for a trouble. Acne will become worse.
- Lemon applied to dry dehydrated skin will burn the skin, causing serious irritation, even though lemon is an excellent option in some other cases.
- In certain cases Salicylic Acid may be added to alcohol and used as a face wash. Great solution. However, Salicylic Acid only works properly if pH is acidic, ideally pH = 3 to 4. It takes a skill to balance the pH level. To accomplish this, glycolic acid could be added, or - even better - resorcinol. This addition makes salicylic acid effective on the skin.

Otherwise it may not work the way it should, or it may even burn the face. So if you heard "salicylic acid" and want to try it on – keep in mind that you heard only a part of the story.

- Sea Salt is often very good, but when blood vessels (capillaries) are too close to the surface, and salt is applied - salt may damage the blood vessels. If this is the case, then baking soda should be used, and not salt. So you would have to make a judgment, it's not enough to borrow an idea from a friend who used sea salt successfully.

- Turmeric is good in many situations, but must be mixed with an appropriate substance first. Otherwise its color may find its way to the skin, and you skin will become yellow. Such a race-changing experience may be socially problematic for you.

How I Anti-Wrinkled My Mother-In-Law

I've been an active skincare professional for 35 years. I've seen it all. Countless faces of all ages and conditions. Untreatable screaming diaper rash. Hysterical teenage acne. Emergency preparing skin for dating. Irresistible beautifying skin for wedding. Pre-pregnancy unexpected acne followed by post-pregnancy unwelcome acne. Beautifying, perfecting adult skin. Reversing shocking early aging signs. Calming down advanced aging skin.

My mother-in-law never paid much attention to my professional life. She had other things to worry about! But suddenly she took an interest in what I do. What happened? She asked questions, but she didn't say directly. I made a guess and called her up. She is 75.

"When did you notice your wrinkles?" I asked.

"Half a year ago."

I was speechless!

"Well, I was told that I had wrinkles a few years before. Over 5 years ago I was at the party, and one of my relatives said that she noticed some wrinkles on my face. I came home, investigated my face for a while, and concluded that she made a mistake. I could find no trace of wrinkles."

"And what happened half a year ago?" I asked.

"I looked in a mirror in the morning, and noticed a light small lonely wrinkle. Not unexpected, but I felt very sad. And now, half a year later, the wrinkles have become more noticeable, so I am wondering if..."

I was surprised. You don't often encounter women who don't have wrinkles till 75. You may ask how I didn't notice this myself, after all I am a skincare professional. But I just didn't. I guess I had other things to worry about :)

Interesting, what if she started using good Anti-Aging skincare when she was 35, would she get wrinkles at 85? 95? Never? I'll never find out...

Naturally, I became curious about her mother, who passed away a few years ago at the age of 90. Our mothers are good indicators about the future of our skin.

"And what about your mother? Did she use skincare?"

"Ugh, My mother... All her life she was militantly against any skincare. She lectured me about it too. I never understood the reasons for her negativity towards it. But shortly after 65, when she got the first wrinkles, she started buying some creams.

Since she was publicly known to be against skincare, she probably felt embarrassed about it, and therefore did it secretly. But I noticed. I found lotions in the oddest places. She kept one in the tea kettle. And then her skin changed a bit."

"Did her skin change a lot?" I asked.

"No, not really, but the difference was enough to notice. This lasted pretty much till the end of her life, so I never had a chance to talk with her openly about it." I could hear a tinge of sadness in my mother-in-law's voice.

I gave my mother-in-law superior products and explained to her how to use them. I was sure the products would drastically change her skin. When I called her some time later, just about when the difference was supposed to manifest, she, surprisingly, wasn't too excited.

"Any changes?" I asked.

"Nah, not much. I see a little bit, the skin has become lighter and wrinkles are less noticeable. The change is recognizable but still very minimal."

I was surprised. The products that I gave her should have produced extraordinary response.

"Do you even use the products I gave you?"

Mothers-in-law!

"Sure!" The tone of her voice made me skeptical.

"Do you use a cleanser?" I was going to give her the fifth degree.

"Well, yeah, I do... Sometimes." And there was the truth! "Often I am not in a mood to take shower at night, so I lie down to read, and become too sleepy."

"Do you use a toner?"

"Well, if I skip the cleanser... I guess I am too lazy or too sleepy."

"What about the night cream?"

"Well, sure, I do... Sometimes. You see, I am not used to it. My whole life skin regimen was never a part of my daily routine, so it's just so hard to incorporate it into my life now. When it's still early in a day - it's too early for it, and when it's already late, I am either sleepy or lazy. But I do use it sometimes!"

P.S. As often in life, it may be easy to achieve results, but you actually have to do it...

Questions? Suggestions?
Comments?

ask@ladore.me

Dora @ LaDore Labs

www.ingramcontent.com/pod-product-compliance
Lightning Source LLC
Chambersburg PA
CBHW070509290526
45790CB00003B/1163